Introduction to Usui Reiki

A COMPLETE GUIDE TO THE HOLISTIC HEALING MODALITY

USUI REIKI – LEVEL 1

Djamel Boucly

© **Copyright 2015 - All rights reserved.**
In no way is it legal to reproduce, duplicate, or transmit any part of this document in either electronic means or in printed format. Recording of this publication is strictly prohibited and any storage of this document is not allowed unless with written permission from the publisher. All rights reserved.

The information provided herein is stated to be truthful and consistent, in that any liability, in terms of inattention or otherwise, by any usage or abuse of any policies, processes, or directions contained within is the solitary and utter responsibility of the recipient reader. Under no circumstances will any legal responsibility or blame be held against the publisher for any reparation, damages, or monetary loss due to the information herein, either directly or indirectly.

Respective authors own all copyrights not held by the publisher.

Author's Disclaimer:
Although Reiki offers a variety of benefits and is practiced all over the world today, the material in this manual should not be considered to override any diagnosis made by a Qualified Doctor or Specialist. But, it can be considered as an additional form of treatment. The author cannot accept any responsibility for any illness arising out of the failure of the reader and/or student, to seek medical advice from a Qualified Doctor or Specialist.

Important note to the Student/Reader:
The purpose of this manual is to offer the reader insight to the teachings and disciplines associated with First Degree Usui Reiki.
The information in this manual has been derived from the traditional teachings of Dr. Mikao Usui and does not contain any of the Authors personal beliefs and or practices.
In order to use this manual to heal yourself or others, you must first receive the necessary Reiki attunements from a Reiki Master.

Table of Contents

Introduction to Reiki 5
   Healing vs Curing 6
What is Reiki and How Does It Work 9
   The History of Reiki 10
   The Benefits of Reiki 15
Reiki Attunements 17
   Before the Reiki Attunement 18
   21 Days Self-Healing 18
   Purification Periods (Healing "Crisis") 19
The Five Precepts of Reiki 22
   For Today Only 22
Self-Discovery – Who am I? 25
   Guides and Angels 29
   Intention is Key 29
Centering and Grounding 31
   Opening Prayer 32
   Closing Prayer 32
   Grounding the Reiki Recipient 33
Body, Mind and Emotions 35
   Overview - Basic Organ Function 36
   Lymphatic System 37
   Body-Mind Connection 39
Human Energy System 41
   Chakras, Meridian System and Aura Anatomy 41
   Root Chakra – Muladhara – *I Am* 43

- Sacral Chakra – Swadhisthana – *I Feel* 45
- Solar Plexus Chakra – Manipura – *I Do* 47
- Heart Chakra – Anahata – *I Love* 49
- Throat Chakra – Visuddha – *I Speak* 51
- Third Eye Chakra – Ajna – *I See* 53
- Crown Chakra – Saharata – *I Understand* 55

The Meridians 59
- Yin 61
- Yang 61

The Human Aura (Energy Field) 63
- A Balanced Aura vs an Imbalanced Aura 67
- The Antahkarana 68
- Spinal Techniques with Reiki and the Antahkarana 68

Self-treatment with Reiki 71
- How to do a Self-Treatment 71
- Preparation for Reiki self-treatment 72
- Standard Self-Treatment Hand Positions 73
- Ending your Reiki self-treatment 81

Treating Others with Reiki 83
- Preparation for Reiki treatment for others 83
- Standard Hand Positions for Treating Others 85
- Position 11 94
- What the Recipient May Experience 96
- Additional Reiki Techniques 98

Final Thoughts 101
- Interesting References 102

Introduction to Reiki

There are various forms of Healing and Healing is approached from various perspectives. Reiki approaches Healing from a Holistic perspective.

Reiki is an Alternative/Holistic form of healing. This means that it does not only focus on healing one aspect (the physical), but multiple aspects such as the body, mind, emotions and the spirit as a whole.

To heal means to "make whole", "to restore to health" or "to restore to a sound state".

Reiki is a Japanese "laying-on" of the hands healing technique, by which the Reiki practitioner serves as a channel to supply life-force energy to the recipient.

This balances the subtle energies within the body and activates the recipient's natural ability to heal body, mind, emotions and spirit.

Healing vs Curing

The word "cure" relates to relief from pain, illness and/or disease and is biochemically based, as it focuses on the physical aspect of the individual and deems a state of good health as a lack of (physical) symptoms.

Whereas the word "heal" means to repair (naturally) in order to restore and maintain the individual's wellbeing. Holistic healing focuses on the body, mind, emotions and the spirit, to determine how each of these aspects plays an integral part in the individual's overall state of wellbeing.

Where the use of modern medication would cure the symptoms of pain or an ailment i.e. headaches, Reiki would be used to heal the underlying cause of the headaches, as it focuses on the body, mind and the spirit.

Taking a pain killer for a headache would cure the symptoms of the headache and the pain would subside in a short period of time. But, the medication is really only alleviating the physical symptoms, not the actual cause.

In the event of regular recurring headaches, healing would consider the origin and/or underlying cause of the headaches. One would then consider whether there are any physical stresses at play, or certain deficiencies within the physical body or possible emotional strain.

Another example would be inflammation. Taking the correct medication and or using the correct ointment to treat inflammation, can surely cure the symptoms thereof. However, looking at it from an energy/holistic perspective, inflammation represents heat and heat represents anger.

One would therefore consider the possibility of an underlying emotional issue. What has possibly caused the individual to become so angry?

Once you embark on your studies of Reiki, you will learn that our emotional state plays an integral part in our overall wellbeing and that stress and an unhealthy way of living can in actual fact be the cause of illness or disease.

Although Reiki offers many benefits and approaches our wellbeing from a holistic perspective (body, mind, emotions and spirit) one cannot dismiss the rightful place of modern medicine.

There are certain instances in which one cannot rely on Reiki alone and where the use of modern medicine is compulsory and unavoidable. Think of a cancer patient in need of chemotherapy. One cannot dismiss this treatment and reply on Reiki alone.

But, Reiki can be used as an additional treatment, which will ultimately help alleviate some of the discomfort and symptoms and provide the patient with a better quality of life.

Reiki can be used in conjunction with modern medicine and is in actual fact offered by many Hospitals today. Some Medical Insurances also cover Reiki Treatments.

CHAPTER 1

What is Reiki and How Does It Work

Reiki ~ is the combination of two words ~ "Rei" meaning Universal Life Force and "Ki" which is Energy. Reiki originated from Japan and was first practiced by Mikao Usui (a Tendai Buddhist Monk/Priest).

In Japan Mikao Usui's healing techniques were called Usui Reiki Ryoho, which means the "Usui System of Natural Healing" in English. This is the system of Reiki which finally made its way to the West and is practiced in many countries all over the world today.

Scientists have done a great deal of research and have proven that the Universe is made up of energy molecules and everything vibrates at either a low or high vibrational frequency, which we observe as "life".

Reiki is a spiritual practice and not a religion. It does not require any form of belief system, in order to be effective. Reiki works on the principle that all is energy. Life energy, which is inherent in all things (in the Universe).

It is this Universal Life Force Energy (within) that connects us to each other, to our surroundings and to the Universe, all forming part of an interconnected unit.

The History of Reiki

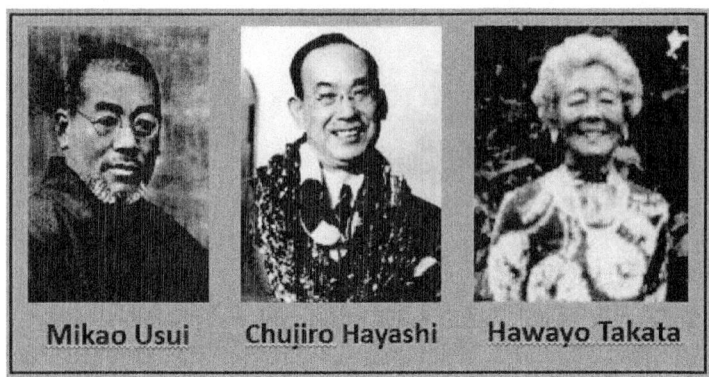

Mikao Usui

Reiki (as we call it today) originated from Mikao Usui, who was born on 15th August 1865 in the village of "Taniai-mura" in the Yamagata district of Gifu region, Kyoto.

It is the assumption of many; that he came from a wealthy family, as only children form wealthy families could obtain a good education at that time.

At a very young age, he attended a Tendai Buddhist Monastery School. He also studied different martial arts. His memorial states that he was talented and hard-working and that he had a vast knowledge of medicine, psychology, fortune telling and theology of religions around the world. This includes the Kyoten (the Buddhist Bible).

He married Sadako and had a son (1907) and a daughter. During the Meiji Era (and later) he travelled to China and western countries several times to study western ways.

He held many different professions during his life, such as public servant, industrialist, reporter, office worker, politician's secretary, supervisor of convicts and missionary. He was also a private secretary to Shimpei Goto, a politician (who was the Secretary of the Railroad, Postmaster General and Secretary of the Interior and State).

He became a Tendai Buddhist Monk/Priest at some stage (otherwise known as a lay priest). He often took a form of meditation, lasting for 21 days. His memorial states that one such meditation took place on Mount Kurama (Horse Saddle Mountain). It is said that this is where he received the inspiration for his system of healing – Reiki.

It is anticipated that he has incorporated his knowledge and ideas about healing from other systems (both spiritual and physical). Such as Chinese Medicine and other Eastern healing systems, like acupuncture, Chi Gong, KiKo (the Japanese equivalent) and others.

He found that the healing techniques within his spiritual system worked effectively on various ailments. He opened his first school/clinic in Harajuku, Tokyo in 1922. He had a small manual, which has been translated into English and was published by Western Reiki Master Frank Arjava Petter, who lives in Japan. It is known as "The Original Reiki Handbook of Dr Mikao Usui".

He must have been a skilled healer and teacher, as word spread quickly throughout Japan. This was a time of great change in Japan. With changes taking place in both Government and Religion and Japan opening up to the West. Older people welcomed his teachings, as they regarded it as a return to old ideals and spiritual practices.

His school not only offered spiritual teachings, but also healing, as people in Japan were very poor at that time. According to history articles healing sessions and other similar practices were either offered for very cheap or for free.

It seems that Reiki students worked with the teacher (as a sort of payment) but a small monetary fee may have been involved.

His teachings also included teaching people how to heal themselves. They would receive healing and be taught how to heal themselves.

On 1st September 1923 an earthquake shook Tokyo and Yokohama. It measured 7.9 on the Richter scale, with the epicentre 50 miles from Tokyo. Over 140,000 deaths were reported. The majority were killed by fires, which had been started by the earthquake. This was the greatest natural disaster in Japanese history. Mikao Usui and his students offered healing in the area and with the great need and demand for Reiki, he became more famous.

In 1925 he had become so busy that he had to open a larger school outside Tokyo, in Nakano. As he travelled a lot, his senior students would continue his work while he was away.

At the age of 62, Dr Mikao Usui passed away on 9th March 1926. He was buried in the Saihoji Temple in Sigunami-Ku, Tokyo. His students later created a large memorial stone next to his grave, with a description of his life and work. A lot of the new information about Usui Sensei comes from the translation of this memorial.

Three levels of teachings

His teachings were divided into six levels, Shoden (4 levels) and Okuden (2 levels) and Shinpi-den. Shoden is the beginning level and the student had to work hard on increasing their own spirituality, before being able to move on to the inner teachings level, Okuden. Not many students reached the level of Shinpi-den, which is Mystery/secret teachings.

It is presumed that he taught his systems of healing to well over 2000 individuals and 15 to 17 individuals, what we call Reiki Masters (but there was no such title in Japan at that time).

Chujiro Hayashi

Dr Hayashi played two important parts in Western Reiki, namely that the hand positions used in the West today, originated from him and that he initiated Mrs Takata to Reiki Master, which brought Reiki to the West.

He was an ex-naval Officer in the Japanese Navy, as well as a Naval Doctor, who graduated Navy School in December 1902.

1925, at age 47, he started his Reiki training with Usui Sensei. He is believed to be one of the last Reiki Masters trained by Mikao Usui.

He left the Usui School after his first training and started a small clinic in Tokyo, "Hayashi Reiki Kenkyu-kai". There were 16 healers and 8 beds. Two practitioners worked together per bed giving treatments to patients.

Hayashi originally used seven to eight hand positions, which covered the upper body only. These positions are based on traditional Eastern healing methods (Chinese Medicine). The "body" is the head and torso and the limbs are considered "external".

When using/treating these positions, which cover the major energy centre's (acupuncture points) the energy will also flow to the arms and legs (using meridians), not only through the body. Therefore, in order to treat the entire body, it is only necessary to treat the head and torso.

Mikao Usui only used head positions and would then treat any other problem area on the body. He also used additional positions for specific conditions.

It is likely that Hayashi may have added further hand positions, which may be the basis for hand positions used in the Western world. These hand positions cover the entire body and enhances the general flow of energy through and around the body.

He compiled his own manual of 40 pages, on how to use these hand positions for specific ailments. He may have given this manual to his students. He initiated about 17 Reiki Masters, including Mrs Takata. Hayashi ended his own life on 10th May 1940, by ritually committing Seppuku'.

Hawayo Takata

Reiki makes its way to the West.

Hawayo Takata was born on 24th December 1900 on the island of Kauai, Hawaii. Her parents were Japanese immigrants and her father worked in the sugar cane fields.

She married Saichi Takata, the bookkeeper of the plantation, where she was employed.

He passed away October 1930, at the age of 34, leaving Hawayo Takata to look after their two daughters. She had to work very hard and with very little rest. After five years she developed a lung condition, severe abdominal pain, and had a nervous breakdown.

Her sister died soon after this and she had to travel to Japan (to where the parents moved), to deliver the news. She also felt that she could receive medical help in Japan, for her poor health. This is where she came in contact with Hayashi's Clinic and received Reiki treatment.

She received treatment twice a day and gradually got better. Within four months she was completely healed. She was impressed with the results and wanted to learn Reiki. She received First Degree Reiki (Shoden) in the spring of 1936. She then worked with Dr Hayashi for one year, before receiving Second Degree Reiki (Okuden).

In 1937 she returned to Hawaii and was soon followed by Dr Hayashi, who came to help her establish Reiki in Hawaii. She was initiated as a Reiki Master by Dr Hayashi in the winter of 1938. She was the thirteenth and also the last Reiki Master that he initiated.

Mrs Takata initiated 22 Reiki Masters between 1970 and 11th December 1980, when she passed away.

These original (twenty-two) teachers also taught others and Reiki has spread rapidly into the East and West since then. Reiki is practiced world-wide and there are thousands of Reiki Masters and millions of people practicing Reiki throughout the world today.

The Benefits of Reiki

- It is a very effective method to reduce stress and enhances relaxation - Thus it enables one to better cope with the daily stresses of life
- It helps to relieve insomnia and aids in better sleep
- It stimulates the immune system, assists the body to release toxins and improves and maintains health
- It removes energy blockages
- It balances and increases the recipient's energy
- It improves concentration and memory and can enhance one's creativity
- It increases awareness
- It relieves pain (i.e. from muscle spam, migraine, arthritis, menstrual pain)
- It brings about a general feeling of well-being
- It calms the mind and the emotions - Thus it brings about a feeling of inner peace and harmony
- Reiki can assist adults, the elderly, children, toddlers, babies and animals

CHAPTER 2

Reiki Attunements

Reiki attunements open and expand the Hara Line (the Ki-holding capacity of the recipient) and clears energy blockages. It opens a channel for Reiki Energy to flow from the practitioner to the recipient.

The more the practitioner uses Reiki, the better he or she is capable of channelling Reiki energy, as the flow becomes clearer and stronger. Reiki is the only Healing art that has the benefit of the attunement process.

A Reiki attunement can be a powerful Spiritual experience, as the attunement energies are channelled from the Reiki Master into the student and this process is guided by the Rei of God-consciousness and makes adjustments according to the need of each student. Reiki guides and other spiritual beings can also be part of and assist in this process.

Some students report having mystical experiences, such as the opening of the third eye, increased intuition and/or awareness, increased psychic sensitivity as well as visions and receiving personal message of healing. Each student can experience something different.

Once you have received a Reiki attunement, Reiki will be part of you for the rest of your life and will not wear off and you will never lose it.

Before the Reiki Attunement

Before receiving a Reiki attunement, you should try to avoid alcohol and/or any other form of drug, as these substances obstruct the flow of Reiki energy.

Ensure to get sufficient rest and try to spend some quiet time or meditate, is possible. Also increase your water intake and avoid eating unhealthy foods. This will assist in keeping your thoughts focused before and during the attunement.

21 Days Self-Healing

After receiving a Reiki attunement, it is recommended that the student undertake a period of 21 days of self-healing. The reasons for this are as follows:

- The Hara line has been opened and because of this, both the energy and physical body are processing and releasing blockages (the system is adjusting). This process takes approximately three days per chakra.
- You will be strengthening your ability to channel Reiki (This takes practice).
- It is said that it takes 21 days to form a new habit. This is a positive habit for the student.

It is important to complete the 21 days Self-Healing. It is advisable to keep a journal during this period of self-healing, to write about your experiences during each healing session.

This will also assist you to better understand and process any past events, feelings and/or emotions that may come to the surface during this period of self-healing. It will also assist you in your personal journey to self-healing, self-love and self-acceptance.

It is also advisable to undertake in regular Self-Healing, in order to maintain your own sense of wellbeing as a Healer.

Purification Periods (Healing "Crisis")

After having received either a Reiki treatment or attunement, there is an increased flow of Reiki within the energy and physical body. This increased flow frees the system of blockages, "toxins" and/or old belief patterns that may have built up within the system over the years.

This purification may result in detoxification symptoms, which one can either experience physically, emotionally or mentally.

These are better described below.

Physical	Mental	Emotional
Headaches	Magnified thought patterns that do not serve	Heightened emotions such as anger or sadness
Cold or flu-like symptoms (i.e. runny nose)	Abusive thoughts or blaming or victimising	
Diarrhoea		
Increased urination		
Temporary skin rash		

When one experiences purification (referred to as "Healing Crisis") the process should not be discontinued, but rather supported. Remember that it is nature's way of healing and release – by bringing these blockages to the surface.

It is important to listen to your body, give yourself time to rest and process. Also ensure to increase your water intake, to ease the process.

These symptoms generally last between two days to a week. However, should these symptoms proceed beyond this time frame, it is advisable to consult your physician, to ensure that there is no other underlying condition causing similar symptoms.

Some do not experience any symptoms of a "Healing Crisis". But you need not be concerned about this, as we all process and release in our own unique way.

CHAPTER 3

The Five Precepts of Reiki

For Today Only

The five precepts of Reiki are spiritual ideals which Reiki Masters and Practitioners can adopt into their daily lives. These precepts bring balance, harmony and more joy into your life.

It assists in living more consciously and to live in gratitude and to appreciate not only what you have, but each and every living being. These precepts also assist you in practicing self-control, as you automatically react differently to various situations which you may have to face. It is a very effective tool to assist you in living more consciously.

Each precept starts with "For today only". The very reason for this is if you falter today, you may try again tomorrow. We are only human, so we make mistakes and improving on oneself is an ongoing process.

You may find days where you do not practice all of the precepts, but therein lays the beauty, that you can begin again anew tomorrow.

"For today only" means that one should not focus on the past, neither on the future; but rather place your focus on today.

- Do not anger – Ikaruna

Do not get angry about trivial things. An example would be someone cutting you off in traffic – instead of losing your temper, think twice about your reaction. Stay calm and do not give your personal power away to anger.

- Do not worry – Shinpai Suna

Do not worry about things you cannot change. If a situation is out of your control, do not spend time and energy worrying about it. Try to turn the situation into a positive, establish what it is that you are able to change and work towards changing it.

- With thankfulness – Kansha Shite

Live with gratitude. Acknowledge all the blessings in your life and be grateful for them. Gratitude creates trust, so trust in the process. The more you practice gratitude, the more you will have to be grateful for.

- Work diligently – Gyo Wo Hageme

Working diligently on yourself. Improving oneself is an ongoing process and you learn something new about yourself each day. Strive each day to work diligently on yourself, to ultimately become the best "you".

- Be kind to others – Hito Ni Shinsetsu Ni

Respect all universal life forces. This includes the spider which landed in your house – he is just lost, instead of killing him, just take him outside. Remember that each living being consists of this universal life force energy.

Chapter 4

Self-Discovery – Who am I?

A universal teaching of all gurus, prophets, masters and avatars is to *"Know Thyself..."*

As you grow in self-awareness and self-acceptance, the better you will be able to understand why you behave a certain way or why you feel the way you do.

By practicing self-awareness and self-acceptance, you will empower yourself to change the aspects of yourself, which you may be unhappy with and ultimately become the "me" that you wish to be.

> *"Knowing others is wisdom, knowing yourself is Enlightenment"* – Lao Tzu

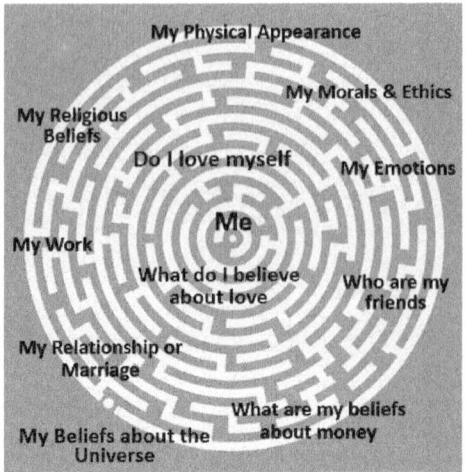

Getting to know oneself is a life-long journey, which will never really end. We all learn new things about ourselves each and every day. When you study Reiki, there will be no exception, as this journey of self-discovery, self-knowledge and self-acceptance is ever-changing and you will discover new aspects about yourself each and every day.

Have you ever really asked yourself "who am I?"

When you strip away whichever title you may hold in your personal capacity i.e. a mother or father, as well as your professional title at your workplace i.e. director or sales assistant - then who are you?

Give this some careful thought and invest in a personal journal for this part of your journey. Make personal notes about "Who am I?" Ask yourself a different question daily, about various aspects of yourself and answer them truthfully.

You may never really finish this exercise, as this is an ongoing process.

Here are some example questions to get you going with this exercise:

- What do I look like (physically)?
- What are my best attributes?
- What do I like least about myself?
- What would I like to change about myself (and why)?
- How can I bring about this change?
- Which emotions are dominant in my life (and why)?
- What makes me feel happy, sad, angry or scared? (List 5 things of each)
- What do I believe about love?
- Why do I believe this?
- Do I love myself? (State why or why not)
- What are my religious/spiritual beliefs?
- Why do I believe this?
- What are my beliefs about the universe?
- Is there anything I would want to change about these beliefs?
- What are my morals and ethics?
- Why are these things important to me?
- What work do I do and do I love my work (State why or why not)
- What is my definition of success (and why)?
- What can I do to change my career or my attitude about my work?
- Am I doing what I am passionate about (State why or why not)?
- What were my parents beliefs about money and what are my beliefs?
- What does money represent to me?
- Do I feel that I earn enough money?
- If not, what can I do to change this?

- What would I do with more money (and why)?
- Who are my friends?
- Do I have many friends (If not, state why)?
- Would I prefer to have more friends (and why)?
- What do my friends and I have in common?
- How do my friends perceive me? (Friendly, realistic, carefree etc.)
- Are my friendships meaningful, if not state why?
- What can I change about this?
- Am I in a happy relationship/marriage? (If not why)?
- What do I perceive as problems in this relationship?
- What can I do to change this?
- What are my partners best qualities (and why)?
- What do I like least about my partner (and why)?
- Will I be happy if my partner does not change?
- What can I change about myself to better our relationship?

You may also add the following questions:

- Do I remember my childhood?
- What are my favourite childhood memories (and why)?
- What did I enjoy doing as a child (and why)?
- Do I still do some of the things I enjoyed as a child? If not, state why?
- What is my favourite pastime (and why)?
- Do I have any hobbies (State what)?
- If not, why do I not have any?
- If I could take up a hobby, what would it be (and why)?
- Do I feel that I spend enough quiet time alone? (If not state why)
- What can I do to change this?

You can add your own questions to this list and remember to be truthful with your answers. This exercise will assist you on your journey to self-knowledge, self-acceptance and ultimately self-healing.

You can refer back to this exercise as often as you feel the need, or as you have time to do so.

Remember getting to know one self is an ongoing journey, so enjoy the process...

Guides and Angels

It is believed that each person has at least two spirit guides, who are always with us and who will stay with us throughout our lives, whether we are aware of them or not; or whether we have contact with them or not. Some may only stay until they have accomplished their purpose.

Not only do they love us, but they are with us to help and guide us and to achieve our purpose in this life. *(Guides have previously had a human experience).*

The notion of working with guides and/or angels is not part of the original Reiki teachings and was added by Western Practitioners. Therefore it is not compulsory to contact spirit guides and/or angels to use Reiki. Your level of Reiki and your ability as a Reiki healer will not be effected if you choose not to use guides or angels – this is your choice.

Intention is Key

As with anything... you should have pure intentions...

To work with intention means to have a purpose or plan in mind or direct the mind to aim. Lacking intention, we may stray without direction or meaning. But, with intention all the forces of the universe can align, to make that which seems impossible, possible.

In the case of healing, it is to have the purpose to heal and this purpose can be directed to another (practitioner-patient relationship), or to one's self.

By grounding and centring one's energy, you can focus and have clear intention to heal.

CHAPTER 5

Centering and Grounding

To become centred means to find quite within oneself and to achieve a focused state. One needs an inner sense of balance (without any scattered thoughts) from which you can connect to the healing energy.

By grounding your energy, it brings you to the "here-and-now" and connects you to the earth's energies. You can use a breathing technique, meditation, visualisation or affirmations to centre yourself.

You can use your own meditation or visualisation to ground and centre yourself or you can use this example:

Sit comfortably with your palms facing up, your eyes closed and breathe deeply (at least four times – breathing in through the nose, exhaling through the mouth).

Visualize that you are standing on a beach. You look down at your feet, the sand is golden brown and it feels soft and warm. You feel your feet gently sinking into the soft, warm sand.

You feel the ocean's breeze gently touching your skin, you smell the ocean and you feel the breeze gently blowing away all your stress and worries.

The sky is clear, a beautiful blue and you feel the sun's rays gently warm your skin. You feel the ocean's waves gently wash over your feet. The water is deep blue and it feels warm.

As the waves pull back into the ocean, you feel all your stress and worries being washed away. You feel peaceful and happy.

Familiarize yourself with your surroundings, regulate your breathing. Now slowly open your eyes and when you're ready familiarize yourself with your surroundings.

Opening Prayer

Sample of an opening prayer:

I call upon my guides, my angles and I call upon Archangel Raphael, the Christ Consciousness, Mother Earth and the Ascended Masters...

I ask that healing energy be channelled through me to... (The recipient's name). I ask that healing take place for the greater good of all concerned.

Let my hands always be hands of healing, to radiate the light, bring about a renewed sense of peace and healing whenever needed.

You can use this example to create your own opening prayer, with which you feel comfortable.

Closing Prayer

Sample of a closing prayer:

I thank my guides, I thank my angles, I thank Archangel Raphael, and I thank the Christ Consciousness, Mother Earth and the Ascended Master.

I am honoured to be a channel for healing, love, light and peace. May the healing continue to take place on... (The recipient's name).

Thank you for allowing me to channel healing, my soul stands before you in gratitude.

Grounding the Reiki Recipient

Spiritual energy is used during a Reiki treatment and just as you have to ground your energy, prior to treating a recipient, you also have to ground the recipient after the treatment, to bring them back "into themselves".

This is reconnecting the "earth" energy and is a very important part of a Reiki treatment.

There are various ways in which you can ground the recipient. You can use these techniques on their own or combine them.

- Use your thumb to press firmly on the Solar Plexus pressure point on the foot (this is just off the ball, at the top of the foot).
- Place your hands on the recipient's knees and gently pull your hands alongside the legs, down to the feet (do this swiftly, but gently) flicking off excess energy, as you get to the feet.
- Offer the recipient a glass of water or a biscuit

- You can also allow the recipient to walk bare-feet.
- You can also allow the recipient to hold a crystal in their hand, but water or something to eat is the fastest way.

CHAPTER 6

Body, Mind and Emotions

You are not required as a Reiki practitioner, to have extensive knowledge of the human anatomy. However, sometimes a basic understanding may be required.

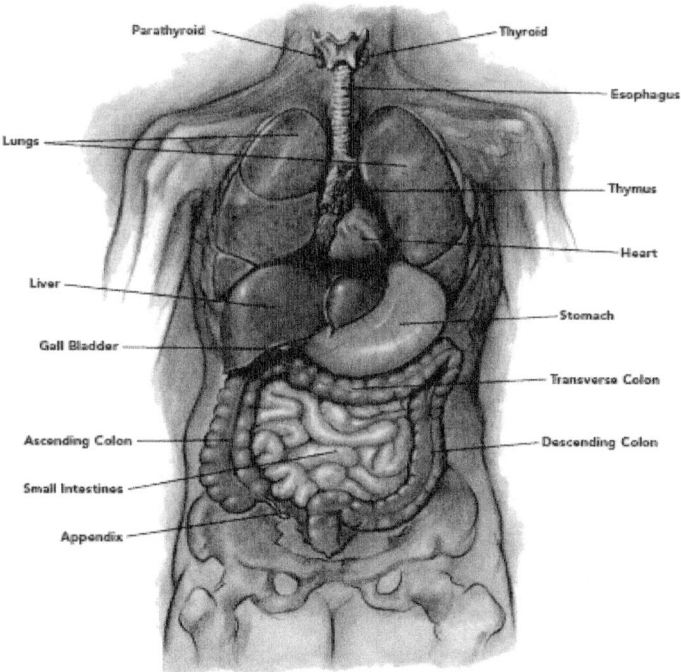

Reiki News Magazine – Front View
Illustration by Tom Bowman

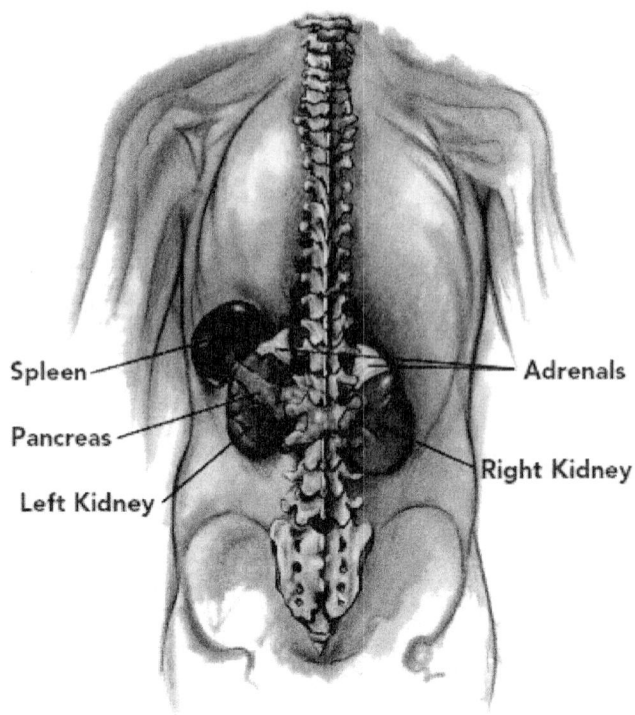

Reiki News Magazine – Back View
Illustration by Tom Bowman

Overview - Basic Organ Function

- Pineal Gland – Located near the centre of the brain (in between the two hemispheres). It excretes serotonin and melatonin.
- Pituitary Gland – Located at the base of the skull between the optic nerves (this is a pea-sized gland). It controls multiple hormonal processes, such as growth, temperature regulation, blood pressure and reproduction etc.
- Parathyroid – Four glands inside the Thyroid. It controls calcium and phosphorus in the body.
- Thyroid – This gland manages metabolism and growth.

- Lungs – The lungs bring life-sustaining oxygen into the body.
- Thymus – This gland is responsible for the immune function and responses in the body.
- Heart – The heart pumps oxygen and nutrient rich blood to and within the bodily organs.
- Liver – This is a multifunctional glandular organ, which filters blood, converts carbohydrates and produces bile.
- Stomach – The stomach holds food and liquids – this is the first stage of digestion.
- Gall Bladder – The gall bladder is connected to the liver and aids digestion, it holds end secretes bile.
- Colon – Also known as the large intestine. Three sectioned – responsible for the final separation of water and nutrients from waste.
- Spleen – Filters foreign matter (infected cells) in the blood. It removes and disintegrates old and/or damaged blood cells.
- Adrenals – These are glands that regulate multiple bodily functions. Best known by adrenaline (the fight or flight response).
- Pancreas – This is a glandular organ which secretes digestive enzymes and hormones. It produces insulin (controls the sugar levels in the body).
- Kidneys – The kidneys separate minerals from toxins in the waste process (urine).

Lymphatic System

The lymphatic system consists of thin tubes, which run throughout the entire body – similar to blood circulation.

The lymphatic system transports lymph (body fluid), which is a colourless liquid and also contains a type of white blood cells, fats and proteins.

Two very important areas of the lymphatic system is the right lymphatic duct, which is responsible for draining lymph fluid from the right side of the body - above the diaphragm down the midline.

The second is the thoracic duct, which is located in the mediastinum of the pleural cavity and is responsible for draining the rest of the body.

It is due to the spleen, thymus, lymph nodes and lymph ducts, that the body is able to fight against infections. The lymphatic system is ultimately responsible for filtering toxins (and germs) out of the body and destroying them.

Body-Mind Connection

Disease and illness are believed to stem from three main areas:

1. Conscious Creation – this is creation by choice (Münchausen)
2. Soul Creation – The universe whispers (conscience), but if not observed it shouts (feelings and emotions), but if not observed, it takes drastic measures (illness or body failure), to persuade you to change your path.
3. Sub-Conscious Creation – 70% of illnesses can be traced back to repetitive thoughts and/or patterns.

Illness or disease can often be traced back to an energetic imbalance or disturbance, whether this is mentally, emotionally or spiritually. Over time, energetic imbalances will manifest into the physical body, either in the form of pain, illness, a deficiency or an emotional breakdown. The result is dis-ease.

There are many excellent books covering this subject and the following books offer extremely helpful insight to the body-mind-connection, how illness manifests and recommendations on how to overcome illness on a body-mind level.

- Your Body Speaks Your Mind by Deb Shapiro
- The Body Has a Mind of Its Own by Sandra and Matthew Blakeslee
- Heal Your Body: A-Z by Louise Hay

CHAPTER 7

Human Energy System

Chakras, Meridian System and Aura Anatomy

Definition of Chakras – This is a Sanskrit (ancient Indian) word meaning "spinning wheel of light". A chakra is an energy centre located within the body and energy filed (also known as the aura). There are seven main chakras within the human body and energy field. These chakras bring energy into the body and also release energy from the body, mind emotions and spirit.

Each chakra has a front and back, the front "feels" – it is charge of feeling and the back is "action" – action is taken from the back. Each chakra has a very specific role.

Something interesting to refer to, are the children's books by the "Grim Brothers", as they all contain a spiritual message. Some examples would be "Snow White and the Seven Dwarfs", "Alice in Wonderland" and "Little Red Riding Hood"

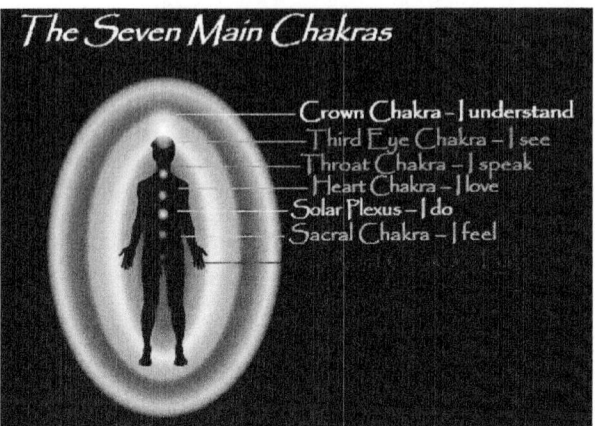

Illustration of the seven main chakras and the aura.
Image obtained from Pixabay (August 2016)

Root Chakra – Muladhara – *I Am*

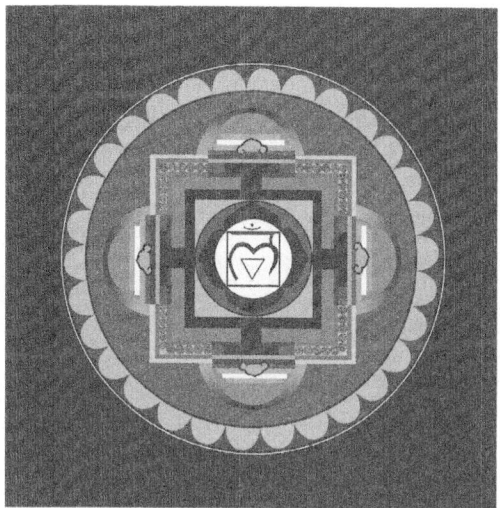

- Location - At the base of the spine/perineum

- Colour – Red

- Element – Earth

- Attributes – Physical body, foundation, grounding, vitality, solidity and survival.

- Bodily Organs – Feet legs, arms, intestines, teeth, nails, anus, rectum cell structure, adrenal glands blood and prostate.

- Development – From conception up to the age of one years old. Babies touch everything (embodiment) and they put things into their mouths (they are learning how to use their bodies). (Trust attachment).

- Notes – Think of Martial Arts – they use chakra energy. The position in which they stand brings the root chakra closer to earth.

Balanced Root Chakra (Muladhara)

When this chakra is balanced we feel optimistic, free, alive, healthy, full of vitality and steady.

Underactive Root Chakra (Muladhara)

When this chakra is not bringing in enough energy, one tends to worry, suffer from anxiety, apathy, lack of will to live and masochistic behaviour.

Overactive Root Chakra (Muladhara)

When this chakra is overactive (brings in too much energy) one tends to feel aggressive, greedy, overbearing and sadistic behaviour – there is extreme and/or overwhelming energy levels.

Sacral Chakra – Swadhisthana – *I Feel*

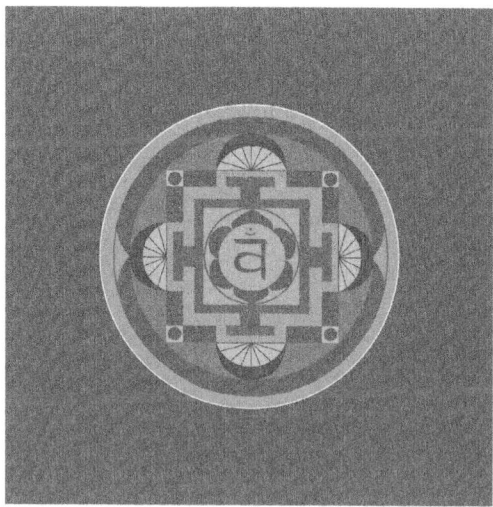

- Location – In the middle between the navel and pelvic bone

- Colour – Orange

- Element – Water

- Attributes – Movement, polarity, reproduction, inner child, creativity, pleasure, sexuality and/or sensuality.

- Bodily Organs – Reproductive organs, bladder, kidneys, pelvic area, sperm – all fluids and liquids in the body.

- Development – Between six and eighteen months. This is when babies start developing their senses (the "energetic growth spurt").

- Notes – This is where the "Inner Child" lives. This is the most important chakra. This period defines our emotions for the rest of our lives.

Balanced Sacral Chakra (Swadhisthana)

When this chakra is balanced we feel creative, open and trusting.

Underactive Sacral Chakra (Swadhisthana)

When this chakra is not bringing in enough energy, one tends to be hyper- sensitive, shy and uncertain, experience feelings of lack of purpose.

Overactive Sacral Chakra (Swadhisthana)

When this chakra is overactive (brings in too much energy) one tends to feel self-absorbed, short-tempered, jealous, as well as feelings of distrust.

Solar Plexus Chakra – Manipura – *I Do*

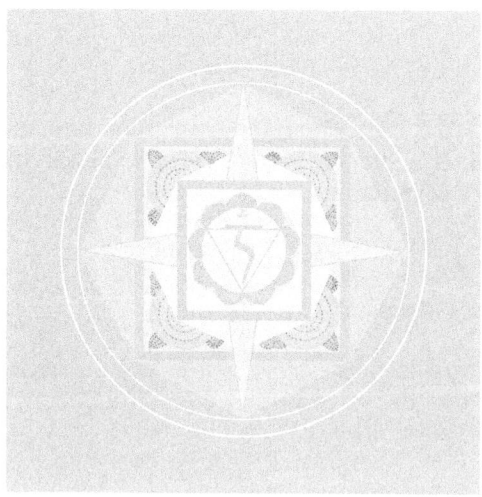

- Location – In the diaphragm area
- Colour – Yellow
- Element – Fire
- Attributes – Power centre, purpose, will, confidence, self-expression and shadow self.
- Bodily Organs – Stomach, digestive system, abdomen, liver, gall bladder, spleen, lower back, pancreas and the autonomic nervous system.
- Development – Between eighteen months and three years. This is when babies start developing a "will centre".
- Notes – This is when toddlers learn to do things for themselves and when they learn about discipline. They learn to control their behaviour.

Balanced Solar Plexus Chakra (Manipura)

When this chakra is balanced we feel happy, confident, safe and powerful.

Underactive Solar Plexus Chakra (Manipura)

When this chakra is not bringing in enough energy, one tends to be judgemental, feel unable to assert oneself, disapproval of oneself and have a fear of authority.

Overactive Solar Plexus Chakra (Manipura)

When this chakra is overactive (brings in too much energy) one tends to feel the need to control, anger, frustration, perfectionism and issues with authority.

Heart Chakra – Anahata – *I Love*

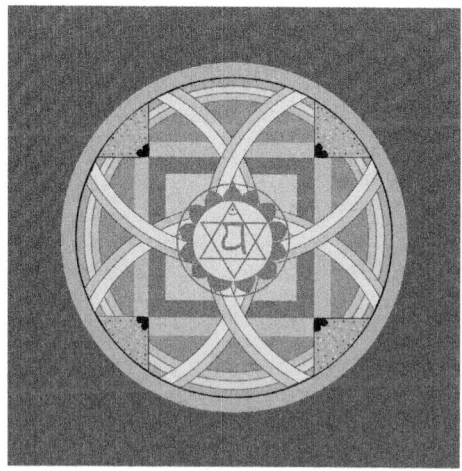

- Location – In the centre of the chest

- Colour – Green/Pink

- Element – Air

- Attributes – Compassion centre, love, balance, joy, surrender, respect, important healing and spiritual centre.

- Bodily Organs – Chest, heart, rib cage, upper back, skin, lower lungs, abdominal cavity, circulatory system, thymus gland.

- Development – Between the ages of four and seven years. This is when we learn to develop feelings/empathy. This is also when sexuality develops. (Even your parent's sexuality is a template for your sexuality).

- Notes – This is where the balance happens. The relationship you have with your mother at this age, will be a template for all your relationships. If this chakra is damaged, it causes damage to empathy and the emotions.

Balanced Heart Chakra (Anahata)

When this chakra is balanced we feel compassion, unconditional love, forgiveness, acceptance and universal trust.

Underactive Heart Chakra (Anahata)

When this chakra is not bringing in enough energy, one tends to experience self-pity, fear or rejection, feelings of being unloved or unworthy, martyrdom.

Overactive Heart Chakra (Anahata)

When this chakra is overactive (brings in too much energy) one tends to be selfish, emotionally manipulating and melodramatic.

Throat Chakra – Visuddha – *I Speak*

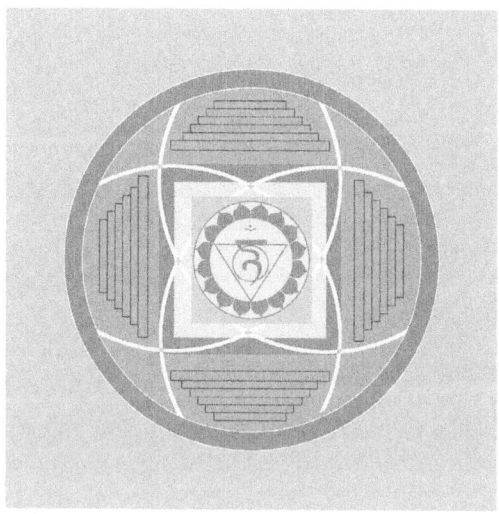

- Location – Between the inner collar bones

- Colour – Light Blue

- Element – Sound

- Attributes – Expression, nourishment centre, creativity, contemplation, ability to relate to others.

- Bodily Organs – Throat, vocal cords, voice, thyroid, thyroid gland, lungs, neck, nape of neck and the jaw.

- Development – Between the ages of seven and twelve years. This is when we start to explore the world. This is when girls get "catty" and boys get "stupid". The ability to create.

- Notes – This is where we learn about the world – the ability to communicate what we want.

Balanced Throat Chakra (Visuddha)

When this chakra is balanced we feel inspired, free, truthful loving communication and self-belief.

Underactive Throat Chakra (Visuddha)

When this chakra is not bringing in enough energy, one tends to experience difficulty of speech, feel introverted and the inability to stand up for oneself.

Overactive Throat Chakra (Visuddha)

When this chakra is overactive (brings in too much energy) one tends to be an excessive talker, domineering, arrogant and the inability to listen.

Third Eye Chakra – Ajna – *I See*

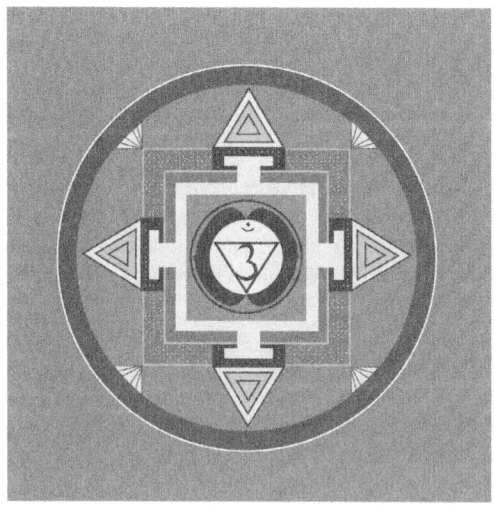

- Location – Between the eyes (also known as the brow chakra)

- Colour – Indigo

- Element – Light

- Attributes – Visualization, wisdom, perception, higher consciousness (intuition), self-awareness.

- Bodily Organs – Eyes, face, nose, sinus, pituitary gland, cerebellum.

- Development – During the teenage years. This is when we start to push every boundary that your parents have set.

- Notes – This chakra is associated with our intuition. This is where we develop our own sense of identity (individuality) and independence. We learn about independence vs responsibility.

Balanced Third Eye Chakra (Ajna)

When this chakra is balanced we experience a feeling of clarity, insightfulness and courage.

Underactive Third Eye Chakra (Ajna)

When this chakra is not bringing in enough energy, one tends to experience a lack of imagination, fear of success and in extreme cases – mental illness.

Overactive Third Eye Chakra (Ajna)

When this chakra is overactive (brings in too much energy) one tends to have a lack of concentration, feelings of confusion and an overactive imagination.

Crown Chakra – Saharata – *I Understand*

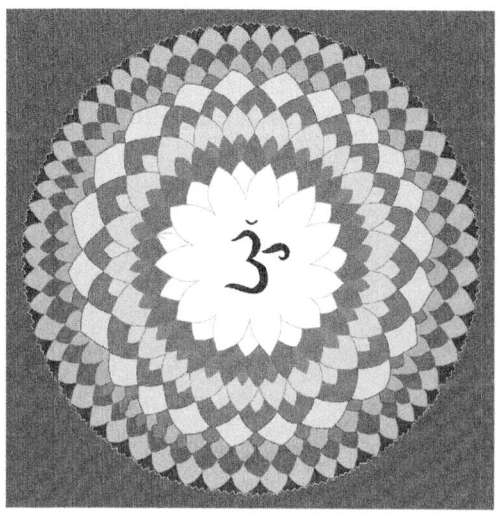

- Location – At the top and centre of the head
- Colour – Violet/White
- Element – Thought
- Attributes – Spiritual centre, direct link to the cosmos consciousness.
- Bodily Organs – Brain, skull, cerebellum and the pineal gland.
- Development – Development starts from about twenty three to age twenty five and continues for the rest of our lives.
- Notes – This is where we start to question everything. This is also normally the period when people enrol for courses (learn) – a time to gain knowledge.

Balanced Crown Chakra (Sasharata)

When this chakra is balanced we experience a feeling of awareness, a deep spiritual connection, a feeling of interconnectedness.

Underactive Crown Chakra (Sasharata)

When this chakra is not bringing in enough energy, one tends to experience a lack of spiritual connection, feelings of separation and a need for control.

Overactive Crown Chakra (Sasharata)

When this chakra is overactive (brings in too much energy) there is a tendency toward extreme religious or spiritual and egotistical behaviour.

The above illustrated Chakra Images are Mandala images – obtained from Pixabay (August 2016)

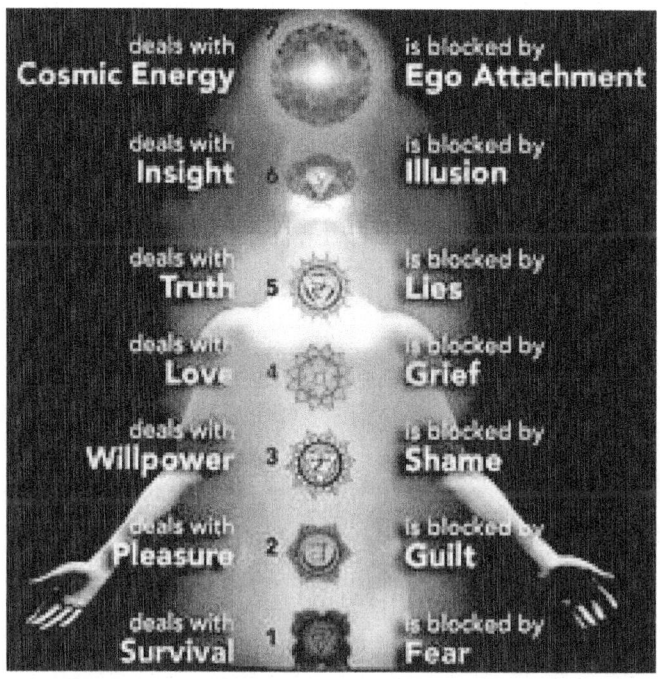

Illustration of Chakras and possible blockages
Image obtained from Pinterest (August 2016)

CHAPTER 8

The Meridians

Imagine that your home's electricity network as a presentation of your body:

- Your chakras are the main power supply, coming in via a supply box, from outside, with multiple transistors which control the flow.
- Your meridians would be the wires (conduits) running through your home (in the walls) supplying electricity to each light, fitting or plug point (which would be your organs, emotional, mental and spiritual functions) in your energy system.

Meridians are the channels through which "Ki" (energy) flows, in order to energise and nourish the body mind and emotions. Meridians also serve as a communication network between the physical and subtle body.

There are twelve main meridians in the human body. Each of them are associated with a particular element and organ system. They are usually listed in Yin/Yang pairs:

This is the masculine and feminine...

Yin – Masculine

Yang - Feminine

- *Metal Element - Lung (arm-yin) and Large Intestine (arm-yang)*
- *Earth Element – Stomach (leg-yang) and Spleen (leg-yin)*
- *Fire Element – Heart (arm-yin) and Small Intestine (arm-yang)*

- Water Element – Bladder (leg-yang) and Kidney (leg-yin)
- Fire Element – Pericardium (arm-yin) and Triple-Warmer (arm-yang)
- Wood Element – Gall Bladder (Leg-yang) and Liver (leg-yin)

The arm-yin meridians flow from the upper body (the torso) along the inner edge (the inside) of the arms to the fingers. The arm-yang meridians flow from the fingers along the outside of the arms to the head. The leg-yang meridians flow from the head, down the upper body (torso) and along the outside or back of the legs, to the toes.

The leg-yin meridians flow from the toes along the inside of the legs, to the upper body (torso).

We experience physical and emotional wellbeing when this flow is unrestricted and balanced. But, when this flow is blocked, irregular or depleted, we experience physical and/or emotional dis-ease.

This information is based on an excerpt from the "Meridian System: Channels of Awareness".

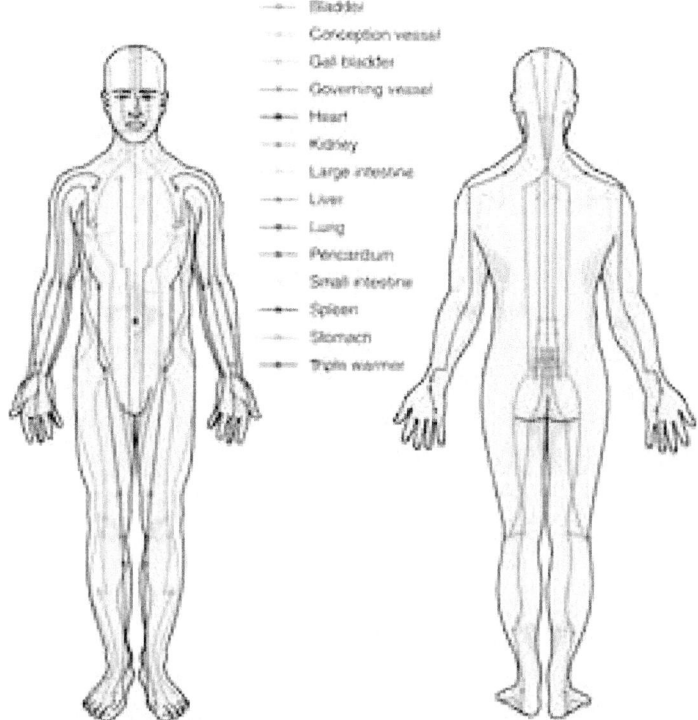

Image obtained from Free Dictionary (Medical Dictionary)

Yin

Yin organs are located deep inside the body and mainly have to deal with manufacturing and storing "Ki" (energy). Yin meridians flow upwards.

Yang

Yang organs are located closer to the surface and mainly deal with receiving, digesting and secreting "Ki" (energy). Yang meridians flow downwards.

CHAPTER 9

The Human Aura (Energy Field)

The human energy field is referred to as the Aura. This is your electromagnetic field, which interacts with the world around you. It is a multi-layered energy system. We will focus on the seven main (most commonly known) layers.

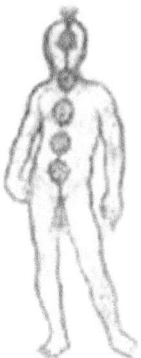

The Etheric Body – The First Layer

This layer relates to the energy flow through the body, via the meridian system. It is 2-5cm away from the body and there is a lot of movement of energy within this layer. You will experience 50% of pain in this layer.

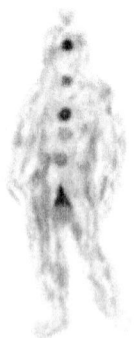

The Emotional Body – The Second Layer

This layer relates to all of your emotions, such as love, joy, anger, sadness etc. This is a fluid body, perpetually changing and moving. The Sacral Chakra defines the color of this layer. It is controlled by an uncontrollable force (and can cause chaos in your body).

The Mental Body – The Third Layer

This layer relates to all thoughts and mental processes and is fed by the Solar Plexus Chakra. When you are doing something that you are passionate about, the Mental Body expands as well. Cancer also starts in this layer.

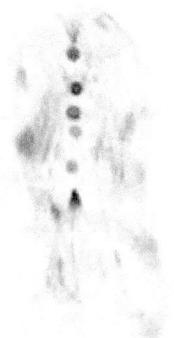

The Astral Body – The Fourth Layer

This layer relates to your connection to the universe and everyone around you. The balance of the physical and spiritual life. This is the layer that connects you to the universe (where your heart strings get attached) and where you distinguish between physical and spiritual.

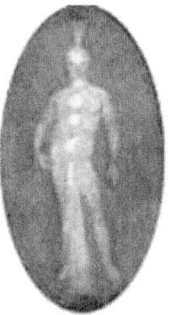

The Etheric Template – The Fifth Layer

This layer relates to your "blueprint" from which you manifested into the physical world. This layer relates to the Throat Chakra. This is where you manifest yourself. This is your soul's plan, what you will look like, the color of your hair and eyes, your build etc.

The Celestial Body – The Sixth Layer

This layer relates to your connection with the divine, i.e. your guides and Angels etc. This is where your soul's emotions are kept. This is also where mother and child are connected. (The Third Eye Chakra).

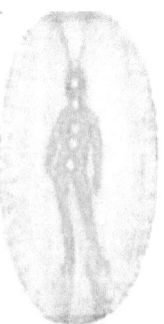

The Casual Body – The Seventh Layer

This layer is also called the Ketheric Template and is the protective energy layer. It provides your energy system with divine protection and love. This layer is connected to your Crown Chakra. This is where your guides and Angels will step in to protect you. When you are being threatened by something or someone this area shuts down like a "trap door". It allows nothing in and nothing out. This layer can be severely damaged by substance (drug) abuse.

A Balanced Aura vs an Imbalanced Aura

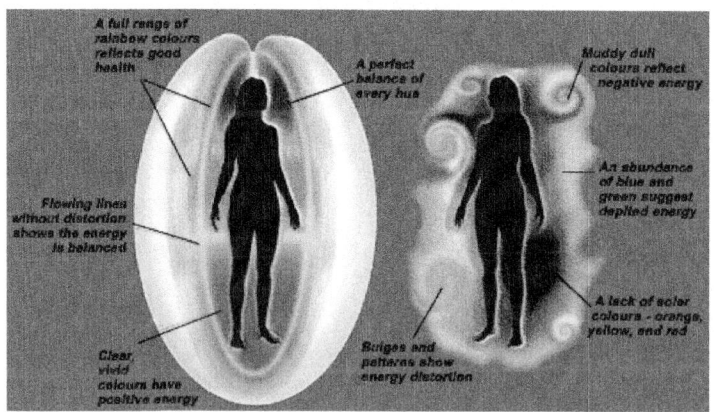

Image obtained from Pinterest (August 2016)

As you can see above, a healthy aura appears vibrant with a lot of bright colours, whereas an imbalanced aura looks dull and appears muddy with distorted colouring.

The aura colours are a reflection (or a "snap-shot") of a person at a specific moment and it constantly changes to reflect the person's inner thoughts and emotions and our thoughts and emotions are ever-changing and evolving.

The Antahkarana

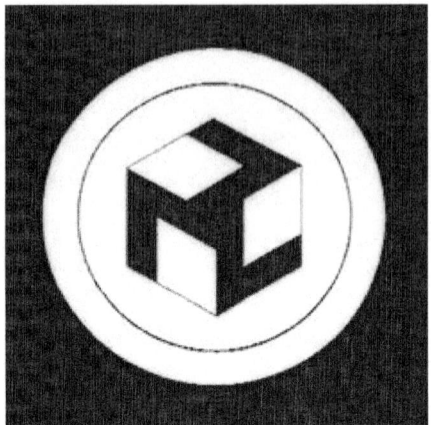

The Antahkarana is an ancient Tibetan Symbol used in healing and meditation.

The definition of Antahkarana:

- Antah – Within (Your actions within)
- Karana – Acting/Action (Your Compassion)

The Antahkarana (also known as) the "three sevens" is a tool which can be used to focus one's attention, thoughts and healing energy. It is believed that it unites the physical brain with the crown chakra. This has a positive effect on all the chakras, meridians and the aura.

The number "seven" is a very powerful and mystical number. It is known as the symbol for movement and energy, as it represents the seven stages or periods of consciousness and transformation.

By placing the Antahkarana in the room where a recipient will receive a Reiki treatment, it focuses and amplifies the Reiki energy and it also assists the Reiki practitioner to remain focused on the recipient during the treatment.

Spinal Techniques with Reiki and the Antahkarana

- The base of the occipital bone has a positive healing charge and can be used in order to relax the spine. Use your left hand as the anchor to link the base to a painful or injured area, using your right hand. This will release blocked energy into the system. This technique can take positive energy into an extremely negative area of the body.

- This technique also works on the navel. Place your left hand on your navel and your right hand on the area where you are experiencing pain or discomfort.

- For pelvic pain – keep your left hand on your navel and place your right hand on the outside of the heel of either foot.

- For urinary, pregnancy, labour or other pelvic conditions place your left hand on your navel and place your right middle finger on the coccyx.

CHAPTER 10

Self-treatment with Reiki

After receiving a Reiki attunement, it is recommended that you undertake a period of 21 days of self-healing.

A self-healing treatment takes approximately one hour. It is therefore advisable to ensure that you have a quiet space available, where you can do the self-treatment.

Also establish what the best time in the day would be for you to do the self-treatment. It is not advisable to do this treatment too late at night, as one may fall asleep if you are too tired.

It is advisable to complete the 21 days of self-healing without any breaks and/or interruptions in between. But, should it happen that you are forced to skip a day or two, ensure to continue the treatments and finish the 21 days.

How to do a Self-Treatment

As you know by now from the section in which we covered the chakras, each chakra has a front and back.

Therefore, you need to focus not only on the front of each chakra (the front of the body), but also the back.

It is standard procedure to spend three minutes on each chakra. However, if you feel the need to spend extra time on a certain chakra or area, it is advisable to do so. Trust you instinct - follow your intuition.

To assist you with the time-keeping during your self-healing treatment, it is advisable to invest in some Reiki music. There are various CD's available as well as downloadable music and free downloads on the internet.

Reiki music generally includes a "bell sound" every three minutes, which serves to remind the practitioner to change hand positions.

Preparation for Reiki self-treatment

- You may wish to create a peaceful atmosphere – light a candle (or two) or burn some incense.
- Centre and ground yourself (by using the grounding meditation).
- Do your opening prayer – you may call on your guides and angels and ask them to assist you to clear the room to assist you with the self-treatment session (Here you will ask for Reiki energy to be channelled through you, to you).
- Make yourself comfortable and begin with your self-treatment session.

Standard Self-Treatment Hand Positions

Position 1

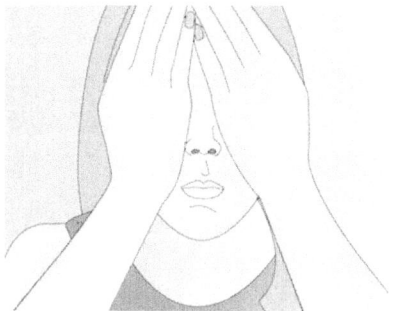

Third Eye/Brow Chakra

Close your eyes and gently place your hands over your eyes. The palms should be directly over the eyes. (Keeping your fingers close together).

Hold your hands in this position for three minutes, using your Reiki music (with the "three minute bell" to guide you when to change positions).

Position 2

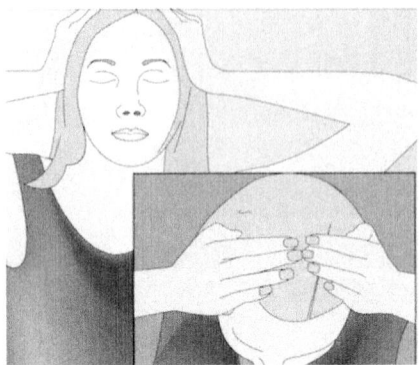

Crown Chakra

Gently place your hands above your ears, (holding your head) with the fingertips touching the crown. (Keeping your fingers close together).

Again, hold your hands in this position for three minutes.

Position 3

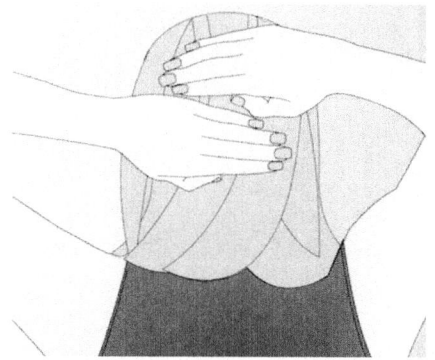

Back of the Third Eye/Brow Chakra

Gently place your hands behind your head. Also ensure that you are seated in a comfortable position.

Again, hold your hands in this position for three minutes.

Position 4

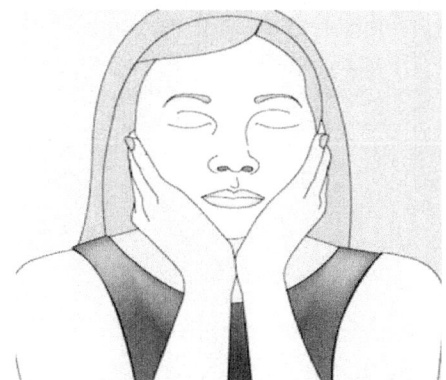

Throat Chakra

Gently place your hands on your face, from the chin upwards (with your fingers gently touching your cheek bones). Your wrists gently touching each other.

Continue to hold each position for three minutes, throughout the self-healing session.

Position 5

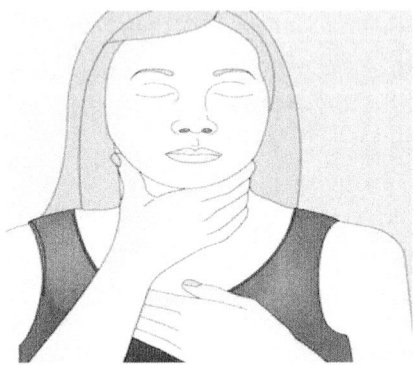

Throat Chakra/Heart Chakra

Gently place your right hand on your throat and your left hand on your chest (over the Heart Chakra).
This position assists one to speak your truth, but with a gentleness from the heart.

Position 6

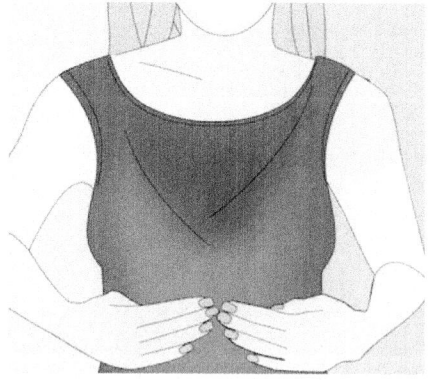

Solar Plexus Chakra
Gently place your hands over your diaphragm area, with your fingertips gently touching each other.

Position 7

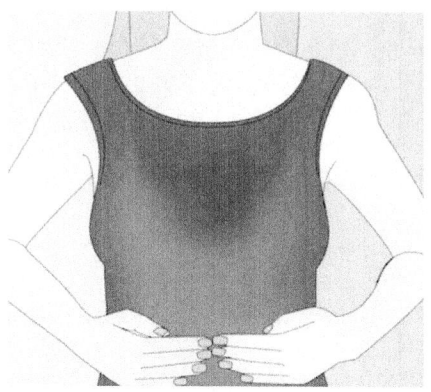

Sacral Chakra

Gently place your hands over the Sacral Chakra (which is located midway between your navel and the pelvic bone. (This is in the area where the reproductive organs are located).

Position 8

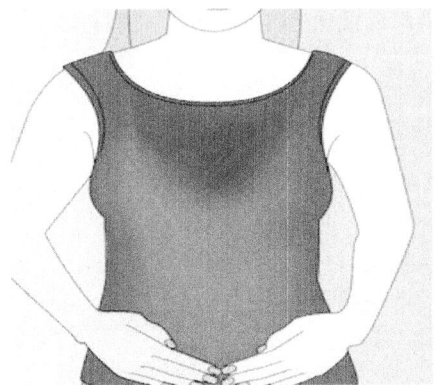

Root Chakra

Gently place your hands in the centre of the lower abdomen - over the reproductive organs (this position is similar to previous position) but focuses on the Root Chakra, located at the base of the spine.

Position 9

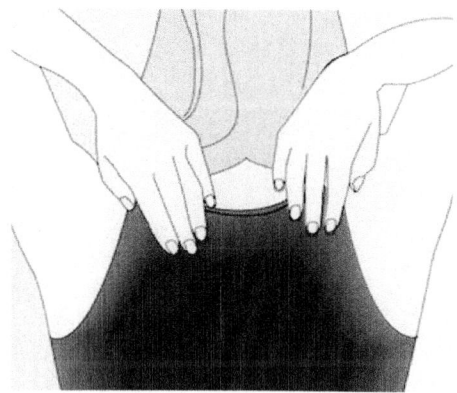

Back of the Throat Chakra

Lift your arms and gently place your hand on the back of your neck, with your fingers touching the top of your shoulder blades.

Position 10

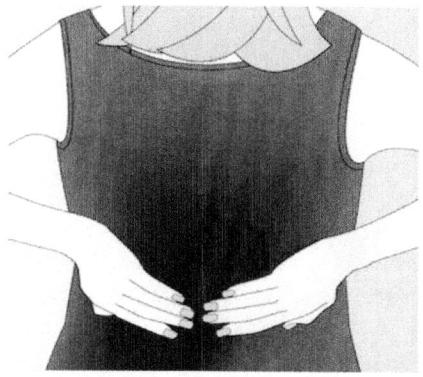

Back of the Solar Plexus Chakra

Bring your arms towards your back and gently place your hands in the centre of your back (at the back of the Solar Plexus Chakra). If you are comfortable in this position, place your hands close together, allowing the fingertips to gently touch each other.

Position 11

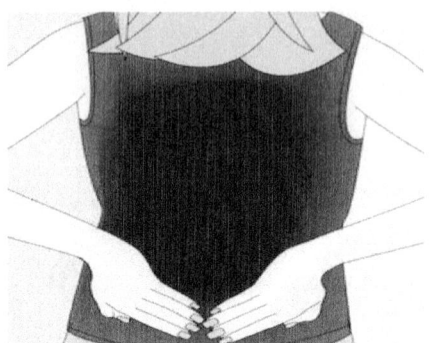

Back of the Sacral Chakra

Lower your arms and gently place your hands on your lower back (just above your hips) – this is the back of the Sacral Chakra. Again, you may place your hands close together, so the fingertips just gently touch each other.

Position 12

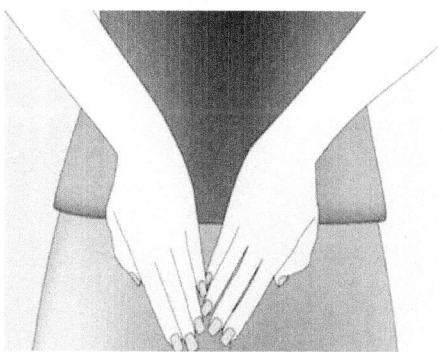

Back of the Root Chakra

With your arms still behind you, lower your hands and gently place them at the base of your spine (just underneath the hip area). Again, you may allow the fingertips to gently touch each other.

Ending your Reiki self-treatment

After completing the last hand position, remember to ground your energy.

- Place your hands on your knees and gently push your hands alongside the legs, down towards the feet (do this swiftly, but gently) flicking off excess energy, as you get to the feet.
- Then sit in a comfortable position, pull your feet towards you (as if in a meditation position) and use your thumbs to press firmly on the Solar Plexus pressure point on both feet (this is just off the ball, at the top of the foot).
- Whilst you are grounding your energy, you may also do your closing prayer.

- Remember to increase your water intake for the following two days, after your self-healing treatment.

- Also remember that you may experience some detoxification symptoms – but if you do not experience anything, this is nothing to be concerned about.

Important points to remember

Remember that there is no "wrong" way of doing a self-healing treatment – Reiki (energy) will go where it needs to go. Always follow your intuition.

CHAPTER 11

Treating Others with Reiki

Although one cannot practice Reiki full-time until the completion of Reiki Level 2, you should practice, in order to enhance both your knowledge and confidence in the overall practice of Reiki.

After completing Reiki Level 1 it is recommended that you practice Reiki on close family or friends.

Preparation for Reiki treatment for others

When practicing Reiki on others, the recipient may either be in a seated position (on a chair). Or you may invest in a therapy bed and allow the recipient to lay down. This is generally more comfortable.

You may also use the therapy bed for your self-treatment sessions.

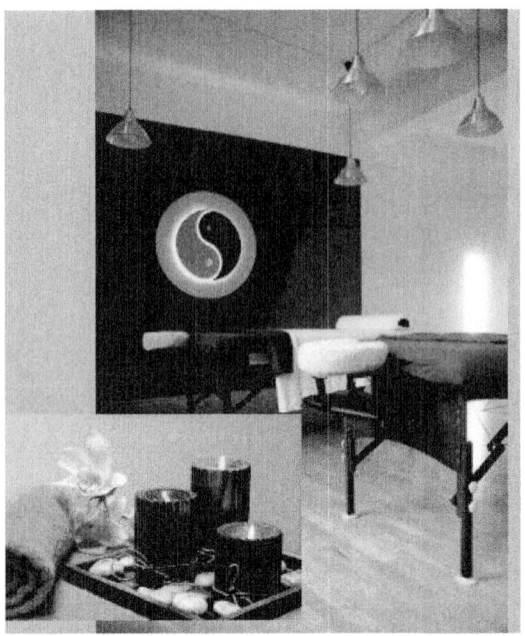

Images obtained from Pixabay (September 2016)

- You may play gentle music or Reiki music (which includes the "three minute bells").
- To create a peaceful atmosphere, you may light a candle or burn some incense.
- Call on your guides or angles and ask them to clear the room.
- Centre and ground yourself (by using the grounding meditation).
- Explain the treatment to the recipient and answer any questions he or she may have.
- Allow the recipient to make him or herself comfortable on the bed.
- Ask the recipient to take a moment, to consciously set the intention to be open to receiving healing.
- Place your one hand on the recipient's shoulder and the other hand on his or her wrist (or elbow). Whilst you are doing this silently do your opening prayer. (Here you can set the intention for healing to take place).
- Then begin with the standard hand positions.

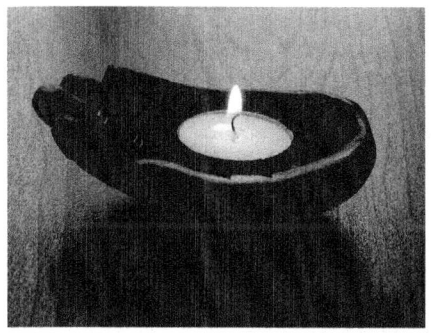

Standard Hand Positions for Treating Others

Position 1

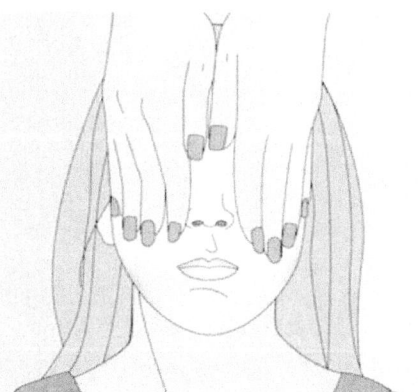

Third Eye/Brow Chakra

Gently place your hands over the recipient's eyes. The palms should be directly over the eyes. (Keeping your fingers close together).

If you are offering a treatment to someone who may not feel comfortable having their eyes covered, you may hold your hands just above the eyes.

Hold your hands in this position for three minutes, using your Reiki music (with the "three minute bell" to guide you when to change positions).

Position 2

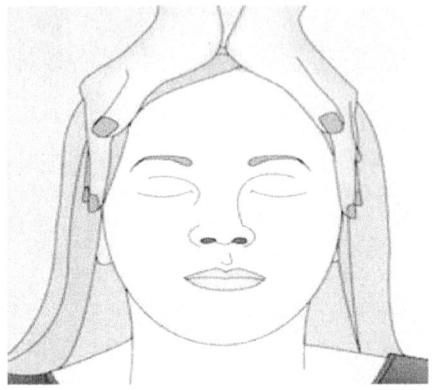

Crown Chakra

Gently place your hands over the top (crown) of the recipient's head, your hands (on either side) with your fingers pointing towards the recipient's ears.

Again, hold your hands in this position for three minutes.

Position 3

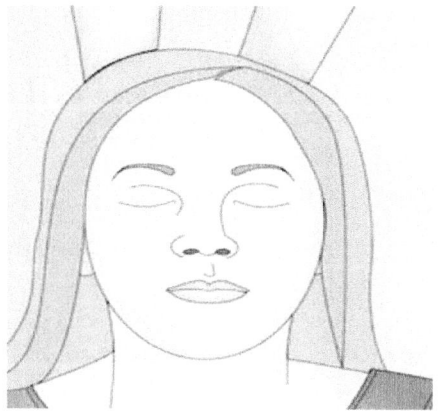

Back of the Third Eye/Brow Chakra

Gently place your hands underneath the recipient's head. (As to allow the person to gently lay their head in your hands).
Remember to hold each position for three minutes.

Position 4

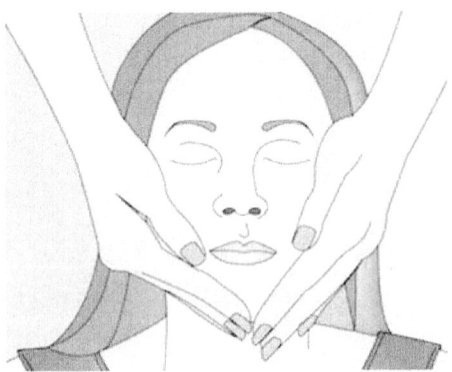

Throat Chakra

Gently place your hands on the sides of the recipient's face, with your fingertips touching at the recipient's chin.
If the recipient is not comfortable having their face touched near the throat area, you may gently place your hands on either side at the collar bone area.

Position 5

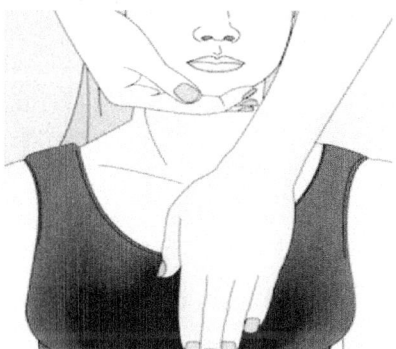

Throat Chakra/Heart Chakra

Gently place your right hand underneath the recipient's chin and the left hand on the chest (on the Heart Chakra).

If the recipient is not comfortable with these hand positions, you may hold both your hands just above the recipient's chest (over the Heart Chakra).

You can place your one hand on top of the other.

Working on the throat and heart chakra will assist the recipient in speaking their truth, but with a gentleness from the heart.

Position 6

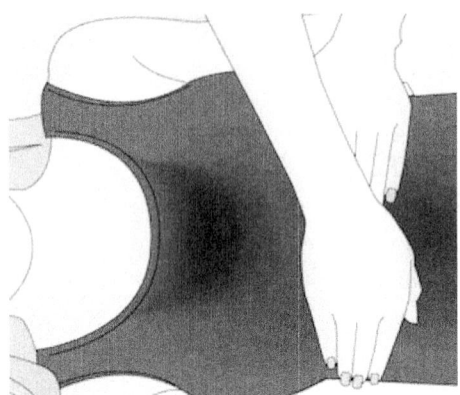

Solar Plexus Chakra

Gently place your hands over the recipient's diaphragm area. Place the hands close together (the one hand may touch the other).

Position 7

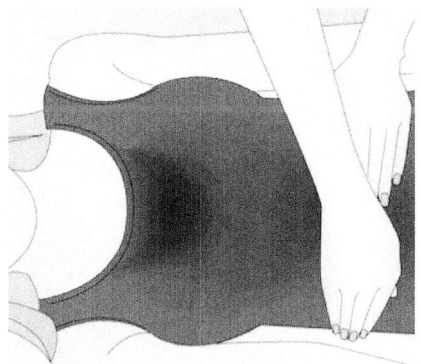

Sacral Chakra

Gently place your hands over the recipient's navel area (slightly above the hip area) over the Sacral Chakra (which is located midway between your navel and the pelvic bone. (This is in the area where the reproductive organs are located).

When offering a Reiki treatment to a male recipient, you may place your hands over the Sacral Chakra, just above the recipient's body.

Position 8

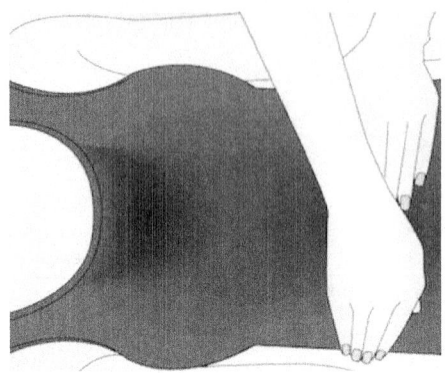

Root Chakra

Position your hands slightly below the recipient's navel area (in the area of the hip bones) - *Keeping your hands just above the recipient's body* (In the area where the reproductive organs are located).

Remember that the Reiki energy will be directed to the area where the Root Chakra is located (at the base of the spine).

In order to proceed to the following position, you will require the recipient to turn over onto their stomach.

Position 9

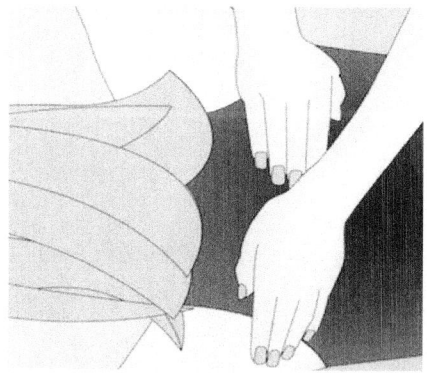

Back of the Heart Chakra

Gently place your hands on the recipient's upper back (in the area just below the arm pits). This is the back of the Heart Chakra. Place the hands close together (the one hand may touch the other).

Position 10

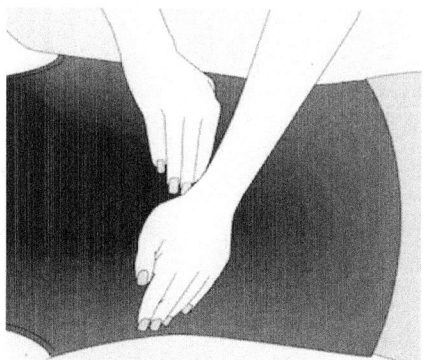

Back of the Solar Plexus Chakra

Gently place your hands in the middle of the recipient's back (in the diaphragm area). Place the hands close together (the one hand may touch the other).

Position 11

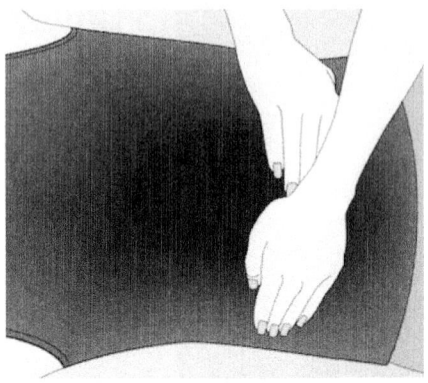

Back of the Sacral Chakra

Gently place your hands on the recipient's lower back, at the navel area (just above the hips) – this is the back of the Sacral Chakra. Again, place your hands close together (the one hand may touch the other).

Position 12

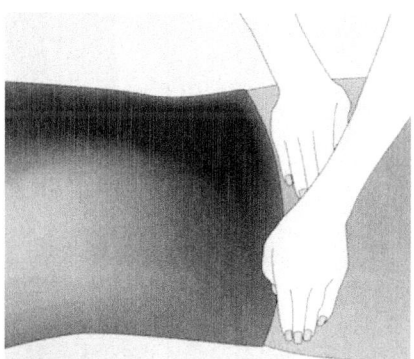

Back of the Root Chakra

Gently place your hands on the recipient's lover back (at the base of the spine (just underneath the hip area). Again, place your hands close together (the one hand may touch the other).

After you have completed the treatment, remember to ground the recipient's energy.

You may do your closing prayer whilst doing this.

You may use one of the following grounding techniques.

Remember that you can use these techniques on their own or combine them.

- Use your thumb to press firmly on the Solar Plexus pressure point on the foot (this is just off the ball, at the top of the foot).
- Place your hands on the recipient's knees and gently pull your hands alongside the legs, down to the feet (do **this** swiftly, but gently) flicking off excess energy, as you get to the feet.
- Offer the recipient a glass of water or a biscuit
- You can also allow the recipient to walk bare-feet.

- You can also allow the recipient to hold a crystal in their hand, but water or something to eat is the fastest way.

Advise the recipient to increase his or her water intake for two days, following the treatment.

You will gain more confidence as your practice Reiki on yourself and others. But to aid yourself in feeling more comfortable with offering Reiki treatments to others, ensure to refer to the "Treatment Checklist" below.

Hand position images obtained from Pinterest (about.com)
Treatment Checklist

- To create a calm atmosphere you may play gentle or Reiki music.
- Light a candle or burn some incense.
- Call on your guides or angels and ask them to assist you in clearing the room.
- Centre and ground yourself (using the grounding meditation).
- Explain the procedure to the recipient and answer any questions he or she may have.
- Allow the recipient to make him or herself comfortable on the bed.
- Ask the recipient to take a moment to consciously set the intention to be open to receiving healing.
- Silently do your opening prayer (whilst doing this, you may put one hand on the recipient's shoulder and one hand on the wrist or elbow). Here you may also set the intention for healing to take place.
- Then begin with the standard hand positions.
- Once you have completed the treatment, ground the recipient's energy (whilst doing your closing prayer).
- You may offer the recipient a glass of water and allow them to leave the room.

Remember to advise the recipient to increase his or her water intake for two days, following the treatment.

What the Recipient May Experience

Not everyone experiences something when receiving a Reiki Treatment. If a recipient reports not having experienced anything, you need not be concerned; as Reiki energy goes where it needs to go and does what it needs to do.

Healing will take place in the area where the Recipient requires healing.

Some recipients may experience the following:

- Some people see colours
- Some people cry – do not be concerned, as this is an emotional release
- Some fall asleep
- Some experience heat
- Some experience cold
- Some experience pins and needles
- Some see images
- Involuntary (muscle) movement
- Some recipients sense the energy (where you may position your hands)
- Some can sense your Guides or Angels

Additional Reiki Techniques

Group Healing

To take part in a group Healing is an excellent way to share Reiki energy. This is also referred to as Reiki Shares. This concept was used by Hayashi in his Reiki centre/clinic.

To be able to partake in a Group Healing, you are required to have at minimum Reiki 1. When doing a Group Healing one person will assume the standard Reiki head positions and the balance of the healers will assume the rest of the positions over the balance of the body.

A group can be made up of 2 to 8 people. Any healers that cannot make contact may stand behind another healer, with their hands on that healer's shoulders.

The flow of energy is drastically increased when there are multiple healers. Group Healing can be a very powerful tool for any recipient who suffers from disease (such as cancer or aids). However, one does not have to suffer from any illness to receive a group treatment.

Chakra Balancing

The purpose of this treatment is to bring opposing chakras into balance. This chakra balance may be used in addition to a standard Reiki treatment.

It may also be used as a brief stand-alone treatment, which lasts approximately 20 minutes.

- To balance the left and right side of the body – place one palm on each foot.

- Place your right palm above the crown chakra and your left palm above the (opposing) root chakra – set the intention to balance these two chakras by using Reiki energy.
- Place your right palm above the sacral chakra and your left palm above the (apposing) third eye chakra – set the intention to balance these two chakras by using Reiki energy.
- Place your right palm above the solar plexus chakra and your left palm above the (opposing) throat chakra – set the intention to balance these two chakras by using Reiki energy.
- Place both hands over the heart chakra and use Reiki energy to balance the chakra. (This chakra is responsible for maintaining balance between the physical and subtle body).

Remember that if you offer this as a stand-alone treatment, you should still follow the steps listed in the "Treatment Checklist" – with the only difference being that you will offer the "Chakra Balancing" instead of Reiki.

There are different variances of Reiki today and one can also offer Reiki Massage, as well as Rei-Flexology (a combination of Reiki and Reflexology).

CONCLUSION

Final Thoughts

- Remember to follow your intuition.
- There is no right or wrong way of doing a Reiki treatment, Reiki energy will do what it needs to do and go where it needs to go.
- Remember that each recipient will experience their Reiki treatment session differently and this is normal.
- Enjoy the journey and enjoy the process.

Reiki is also effective on the following:

- Your computer
- Your home and your car
- A flat car battery
- Your food
- Your plants
- Your pets
- Your drink water (or bath water)
- You can use Reiki at your work
- You can use Reiki for protection while travelling

Once you have been attuned to Reiki, it will always be a part of you, whether you studied Reiki for self-growth only, or wish to open your own practice.

Each Reiki Master, student/practitioner has his or her own unique gift. Those who require your gift will be guided to find you.

Interesting References

Once one opens up to the concept that "all is energy" and you commence with studies such as Reiki Healing, it opens up to us a cosmic journey of growth, self-love, self-acceptance and ultimately self-healing.

There are various books and resources available, offering valuable insight and information about Reiki and energy.

Below is a list of books you may find resourceful.

The Spirit of Reiki
W. Lubeck, F. Arjava Petter & W. Rand

Hands of Light
Barbara Ann Brennan

The Reiki Source Book
Bronwen & Frans Steine

Light Emerging
Barbara Ann Brennan

Wheels of Light
Rosalyn Bruyere

On your journey of self-discovery and self-healing, you may also find the following books helpful.

A Step in the Right Direction – Daily Devotional
Jennifer Rossouw
(A spiritual devotional with inspirational messages for each day of the year)

The Alchemist
Paulo Coelho
(About learning the language of the universe)

The Teachings of Lao Tzu – The Tao Te Ching

Translated by Paul Carus
(A valuable guide about the teachings of Lao Tzu)

Angel Therapy
Doreen Virtue Ph.D.
(This book is a valuable guide through difficult times)

Sixth Sense
Stuart Wilde
(This book is a valuable guide to using your intuition)

The Crystal Bible Volume 1
Judy Hall
(A valuable guide to over 200 crystals) – Although there are later versions available today

Your Body Speaks Your Mind
Deb Shapiro
(About the association between body and mind)

Printed in Great Britain
by Amazon